W0017846

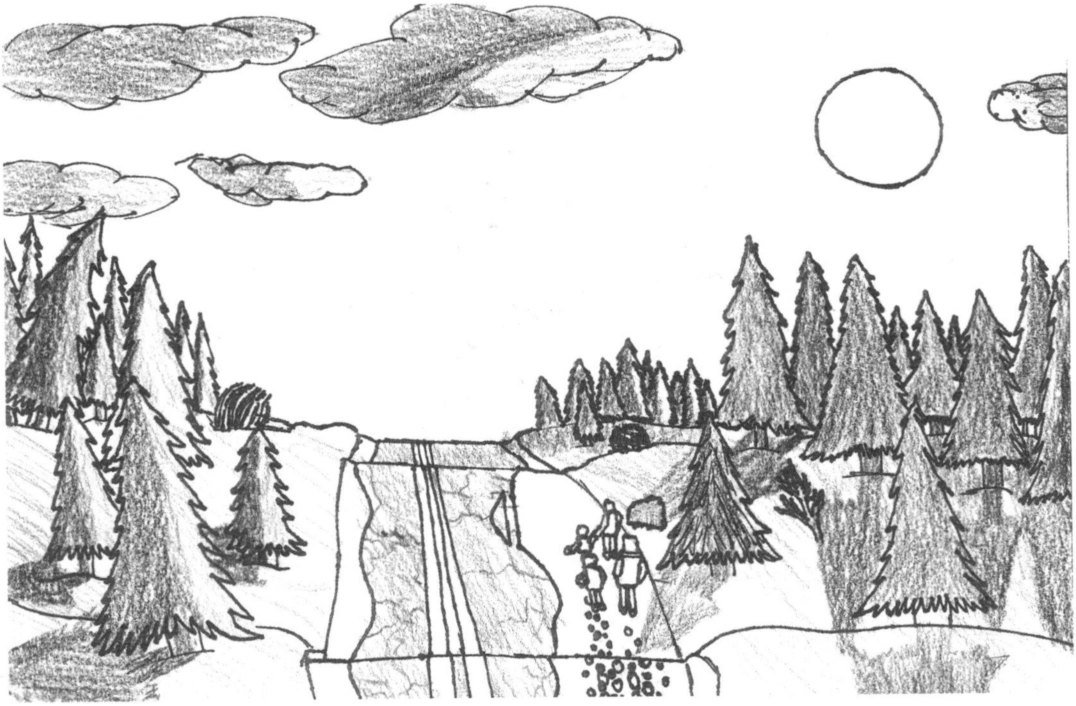

Rose Swallow odibaajimowin imaa Chisaasibiing
The Story of Rose Swallow of Chisasibi

Told by Rose Swallow
Written by Ruth DyckFehderau
Translated into Ojibwe by Patricia M. Ningewance

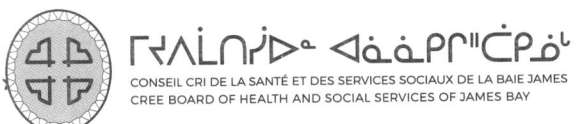

ᒥᐢᐱᒫᑎᓯᐎᐣ ᐊᐧᐊᐧᐱᕆᐦᑖᐳᐧᐧ
CONSEIL CRI DE LA SANTÉ ET DES SERVICES SOCIAUX DE LA BAIE JAMES
CREE BOARD OF HEALTH AND SOCIAL SERVICES OF JAMES BAY

Funding for this publication was provided in part by Health Canada. The opinions expressed in this publication are those of the storyteller and do not necessarily reflect the official views of Health Canada or of the Cree Board of Health and Social Services of James Bay.

Some names and details in this book may have been changed for the purpose of protecting identities. Any similarities between these changed names or details and real persons, living or dead, is not intended.

First printing, 2020. Printed and bound in Canada by Houghton Boston Printers, Saskatoon, Saskatchewan. Distributed by Wilfrid Laurier University Press / wlupress.wlu.ca

Set in Verdana font, chosen for its readability. Printed on paper that is Forest Stewardship Council-certified with post-consumer recycled fibres, and that is acid- and chlorine-free.

Cover design by Nicole Ritzer, based on an original design by Cameron Mosimann. Photograph of Mistissini burnt forest (reversed) taken by Davic DyckFehderau. Title page illustration by Jarred Voyageur of Mikw Chiyâm Arts Concentration Program, Voyageur Memorial High School, Mistissini, QC.

All rights reserved. The use of any part of this publication, reproduced, stored in a retrieval system, or transmitted in any form or by any means (electronic, mechanical, photocopying, recording, or otherwise) without prior consent is an infringement of copyright law. Contact Cree Board of Health and Social Services of James Bay for further details.

Copyright © 2020 Cree Board of Health and Social Services of James Bay
Published by Cree Board of Health and Social Services of James Bay
Contact: Paul Linton, 168 Main St, Mistissini, QC, Canada, G0W 1C0 / (418) 923-3355
creehealth.org / sweetbloods.org

Library and Archives Canada Cataloguing in Publication

Title: Rose Swallow odibaajimowin imaa Chisaasibiing = The story of Rose Swallow of Chisasibi / written, Ruth DyckFehderau o-gii-ozhibii'aan ; told, Rose Swallow ; translated into Ojibwe, Patricia M. Ningewance.

Other titles: Story of Rose Swallow of Chisasibi

Names: DyckFehderau, Ruth, author. | Container of (work): DyckFehderau, Ruth. Story of Rose Swallow of Chisasibi. | Container of (expression): DyckFehderau, Ruth. Story of Rose Swallow of Chisasibi. Ojibwa. | Cree Board of Health and Social Services of James Bay, publisher.

Description: "A Story from The Sweet Bloods of Eeyou Istchee: Stories of Diabetes and the James Bay Cree." | Text in Ojibwa and English.

Identifiers: Canadiana 20200218751 | ISBN 9780973054293 (softcover)

Subjects: LCSH: Swallow, Rose. | LCSH: Diabetics—Cree Nation of Chisasibi—Biography. | LCSH: Diabetes—Cree Nation of Chisasibi. | LCGFT: Biographies.

Classification: LCC RC660 .D96 2020 | DDC 362.1964/620092—dc23

Gii-ikwezensiwipan Rose, gaamashi gikino'amaadiiwigamigong gii-ayaasii iwe apii, omishoomisan o-gii-wiijiiwaan wedi Gichi-ziibiing e-gii-izhaawaad ji-naadisabiiwaad. Gii-gichi-giizhoopizowag. Animosha' o-gii-odaaba'aawaa' imaa gichi-wiikwedong Hudson Bay gaa-izhinikaadeg. Wiin wiin Rose gii-bimidaabaazo, wiinge ishpaagwanagaanig, e-gizhaateg gaye gii-gizhebaawagak. Gichi-bimiba'idiwag igi animoog, omishoomisan dash bimibatoowan jiigi-daabaanaak. Ngoding ako ogijigwaashkwani imaa odaabaanaakong ji-anwebid ajina.

"Inashke!" odinaan oozhisan, "Inashke epiichi-gagiitaawendamowaad igi animoog. O-gikendaanaawaa aaniindi ezhi-naniizaanadaninig, ezhi-bibagizhezigwaag amii dash imaa gaawiin izhaasiiwag. Ogikendaanaawaa. Bizaanigo gidizhaamin ebiwaad nindasabiig gaa-izhi-gizhiijiwang ziibi, nawach naniizaanizi mikom, wiinawaa dash ogikendaanaawaa aaniindi ge-izhaasigwaa."

Gaawiin dash wii-ayeko'aasii' oda'isha, e-gozigonid wiin. Gii-gabaagwaashkwani wiiba, miinawaa e-bimibatood.

Gii-odisaawaad bezhig asabiin, Rose gii-gabaa. Gii-anweshinoog dash igi animoog. Omishoomisan dash gii-naadisabiibani'owan. Gozigwani a'a asab e-bida'anaad giigooya'. Gichi-gaanjitaa

When Rose was a young girl, not yet in school, she and her grandfather swaddled against the cold bay wind and took the dogsled over Hudson Bay and up the La Grande River to check the fishnets. Rose perched up on the sled, the sun glinted off snowdrifts around her, the frenzied huskies kicked up snow in front of her, and her grandfather ran alongside the sled. Sometimes he jumped on for a minute or two of rest.

"Look," he said then, "you can see how smart the dogs are. They know where the ice is thin and they avoid it. We can go to my river nets, where the water runs faster and the ice is more dangerous, only because of them."

He didn't want to tire the huskies with his extra weight, though, and soon hopped off the sled again to lope along beside.

When they reached a fishnet, Rose climbed down from the sled and the dogs rested while her grandfather, after all that running, heaved up the catch. The net was so heavy with ice and water and fish e-zaagijidaabiid ini giigooya' epiichi-gozigoninid. Wewiib ogijigonaa' imaa asabiing ebakitewaad giishpin giiyaabi bimaadizinid. O-gii-dakobinaa' dash imaa, odaabaanaakong o-gii-asaa'. Aazha miinawaa boozi Rose. Apane miinawaa godag asabiin enaanzikawaawaad.

Gii-onaagoshininig gii-ayaawaad waakaa'iganensing, o-gii-giizhideboonaa' animoo' omishoomisan, okanan gaye wiiyaas gaye manoomin.

"Weweni gi-daa-ashamaag animoog," odigoon, "Endaso-giizhig, niizhing endaso-giizhig, gaawiin gaye eta gii-odaabiiwaad. Gego wiikaa maanzhidoodawaaken animosh. Weweni doodaw."

Baamaa gaa-ishkwaa-wiisiniwaad animoshag gaa-izhi-onabid wiin, e-wiisinid.

Gii-niibininig, gii-giigooyikaanig, owiiji'aan ako ookoman Rose e-ozhitoowaad agwaawaanaak. Mitigoonsa' odaabaji'aawaa', gaye ojiitadeyaab. Gii-giizhitoowaad boodawewag imaa, gaa-zhakaakwag mishi odaabajitoonaawaa ji-gichi-biskanesinog. Amii dash imaa ezhi-agoonaawaad giigoowa' gaa-ishkwaa-baanizhwaawaad. Gabe-giizhig baasowag. Amii dash bagwaanishing ezhi-gashkiiginaawaad, mashkimoding

that his body leaned back on an angle and his arms and legs strained with the weight of it. He untangled the fish from the net, bashed them on the ice to kill them quickly, bundled them and lashed the bundle to the sled. Rose climbed back on top of the load, and they were off again, on to the next net, grandfather running beside.

Back at the cabin at the end of the day, her grandfather cooked up a big meal with bones and meat and rice for the dogs.

"You must feed dogs well," he said. "Every day, twice a day, and not only on the days they pull the sled. Never be cruel to a dog; you have to respect each one."

Only after the dogs were fed did he sit down himself and rest.

In the summers, when fish were more plentiful, Rose helped her grandmother build a drying rack from saplings and sinew. They straddled it across a damp-wood fire and together they draped fish over the rack to smoke until they were well-preserved. They wrapped the fish up in a cloth from a flour sack and loaded the bundles into sacks. Then they carted the sacks on their backs to her grandmother's cache, a storage area 15 minutes away

2

ezhi-biinawaawaad. Amii dash ezhi-bimiwanewaad waanikaaning ji-izhi-asanjigowaad. Aki aasaakamig imaa o-gii-atoon ji-onji-dakiziwaad igi giigooyag gaa-baasowaad. Gaawiin dash da-onaajishinziiwag niibing gizhideg. Gaa-ishkwaa-ningowaawaad amii ezhi-asaawaad gaa-gozigoninid asinii' ogijiya'ii ji-waanikesigwaa ma'iinganag.

Aya'aawishensa' daabishkoo bineg gaye waaboozoog onisaawaa' gaye gaa-mindidowaad daabishkoo moonzoog adikwag emitosewaad omishoomisan gaye ookoman, maagizhaa gaye enagwaanaawaad ewanii'igewaad. Gii-ishkwaa-naawakwenig ako ookoman Rose owanzaan wiiyaas boodawaanaabikong, bakwezhiganaabo e-ozhitood gemaa naadowensa'. Oodenaang odoondinaawaan ini biisadaawang bakwezhiganan. Gii-baatiinod bakwezhiganike ko.

Mawinzowag ngojigo miinigiizis gii-bimangizod, gii-miinikaag iwe apii. Wiinge ko gichi-mawinzowag gii-ishkwaa-naawakwenig. Baashkiminisigewan ookoman, gemaa zhiiwi-bakwezhiganing odasaa'. Amii dash gaye gaa-izhichiged e-gii-baasang ini miinan mashkimoding dash ebiina'ang gaawiin dash wanaadanzinoonan. Amii dash ako gabe-biboon e-ayaawaad niibiwa miijim ge-miijiwaad.

that she had dug out underground and lined with moss for insulation. They placed the fish bundles inside the moss where they would stay cool and piled on top the heaviest rocks they could find so the wolves couldn't get at them.

The big and small game – moose and caribou and grouse and rabbit – was all hunted on foot, or caught in snares and traps that her grandparents would walk to every week. Over long afternoons, Rose's grandmother would slow-cook the game into stews and float soft dumplings in the dark gravies. The flour had been purchased in town and sometimes, when there was enough of it, she made bannock to sop up the juices.

Berry-picking time came around August, when the blueberries were a deep navy and had sweetened in the sun. Rose and her grandparents walked out in the afternoons and picked all they could find. Her grandmother boiled some berries into jams or folded them into cakes, and the rest she dried and preserved in a cotton bag where they wouldn't mould. And with the fish and the berries and other hunted meats, they had food in the long winter months.

Ngoding gii-maneziwag miijim. Aanawi gii-ozhitoowaad miijim gii-niibininig ge-miijiwaad biibooninig giiyaabi ko gii-jaagisewag. Amii ko wedi minising wiikwedong ezhaanid Rose omishoomisan enaanzikamonid waakon. Nitaawigin imaa ogidaabik. Makadewaa daabishkoo gichi-aniibiish gaa-adaaweng adaawewigamigong izhinaagwan. Wanzigaadeg bizaanigo gi-miijin. Amii gaa-miijiwaad awiyag ji-gawaskadesigwaa mewinzha.

Gii-gichi-anokiiwag mewinzha awiyag ji-bimaadiziwaad, ji-ondinamowaad ge-miijiwaad. Apane go gii anokiiwag. Gaawiin dash wiikaa awiya gii-ziizibaakwadwaapinesii iwe apii.

Ango-biboon gaa-izhiseg gii-wiijiiwaapan omishoomisan Rose enaadisabiinid, gii-namadabi gikino'amaadiiwigamigong e-ganawaabandang gegoon odoonaaganing. Broccoli odizhinikaadaanaawaa igi wemitigoozhii-gikino'amaagewikweg. Gii-inaa ji-miijid gaawiin dash miijim odinendanziin. Oganawaabamigoo'. Giishpin miijisig o-da-bakite'ogoo'. Gemaa gaawiin da-ashamaasii miijim. Ezhi-gashkanzagwaabid enaanaagadawendang gegoon gaa-zaagitood daabishkoo gii-gikino'amawind ji-baakwaa'ishiimod gemaa ji-bakwezhiganiked. Izhi-daawani ebakiindang iweni broccoli. Omaanzhipidaan. Ozhaashaagwandaan.

Some years, the years of starving, were bad. Even with the fishing and the hunting and the berry-picking, there wasn't enough food. Then Rose's grandfather would go out to the islands in the bay. There was a lichen that grew there; it was something like a black moss and something like lettuce. You could boil it, if you had to, and eat it. It would get you through the bad times.

It was an athletic life, living on the land. You were always moving, just to be able to eat. Always doing something. No one in the area had heard of diabetes then.

The year after the dogsled rides to the fishnets, Rose sat in the residential school dining room contemplating something on her plate. The teachers called it "broccoli" and Rose was supposed to eat it – but it didn't look like food. She was being watched, though: if she didn't clean her plate she would be punished and either starved or beaten until she couldn't get out of bed. And so she closed her eyes, tried to think about the parts of her school day that she enjoyed – like French class and baking class and handicrafts – and she stabbed her fork into that vile broccoli stem and willed her mouth to open. When she closed it, bitter juices squirted across her tongue and in seconds

Onoondawaa' godag abinoojiizha'
e-aa'aagadenid e-gagwe-miijinid iweni
broccoli. Nawach maawiin maanzhipogwan
owe broccoli apiich wiin waakon inendam.
Amii sa gaa-izhi-gidaanawed. Gichi-
ayaawiyaan ayaawagwaa abinoojiizhag
gaawiikaa nin-ga-ashamaasiig broccoli
inendam. Iwe apii gaawiin mashi awiya
gii-ziizibaakwadwaapinesii.

Ngoji go 1960 gii-izhisenig biindige
gaa-izhi-zaaga'amowaad ikwezensag
imaa ishpi-gikino'amaadiiwigamigong
imaa Rouyn-Noranda. Bezhig ikwezens
imaa niibawi. Odishpiiginaan ogoodaas,
amii dash ezhi-jiita'odizod zhaabonigan
e-aabajitood, mashkiki e-miinindizod.
Gaa-minwendamoshkaagemagak
mashkiki odaabajitoon, odinenimaan.
Maamakaadendam Rose. Gii-giziininjii,
amii dash gaa-izhi-maajaad. Gaawiin
gegoon odinaasiin. Eniizho-biboonagaak
dash Biology gaa-izhinikaadeg
gikendaasowining odizhi-bizindawaan
gikino'amaagewikwen e-dazhindaminid
ziizibaakwadwaapinewin, e-jiita'odizowaad
dash iwe gaa-inaapinewaad.
Omikwenimaan ini ikwezensan gaa-
gii-waabamaapan e-jiita'odizonid. Amii
ngwana nitam e-gii-waabamaad awiyan
iwe e-inaapinenid.

Ogii-giizhitoon ogikino'amaagoowin
Rose, gii-anokii dash imaa Jizaasabii
HBC adaawewigamigong. Ngojigo 1970

the broccoli became a revolting mush. All
around her in the dining room, Cree kids
were gagging and vomiting at the strange
food. This had to be worse than that black
lichen her grandparents had eaten in the
starving times. But Rose forced it down
and avoided a beating. *When I grow up*,
she thought, *I will have kids. And I will
never force them to eat broccoli.* In those
years, there was still no talk of diabetes.

In the late '60s, Rose walked into the
bathroom of her high school in Rouyn-
Noranda. Another student was there: a
girl who had hiked up her skirt, propped
her leg up on the big round water fountain
– and was sliding a needle into the flesh
of her thigh. *A heroin addict,* thought
Rose, *right here, in my high school!* Rose
washed her hands at the fountain and
returned to class without saying anything
to the girl. A few years later, though, in
Biology class, the girl came to mind again.
The teacher talked about the pancreas
and a disease called diabetes which was
treated with injections of insulin. That
needle girl had been injecting not heroin
but insulin, Rose realized, and without it
she would have died. She was the first
person with diabetes that Rose ever saw.

Rose finished her schooling and found
work at the Chisasibi Hudson's Bay Store.
It was the '70s, a time of big changes.

gii-izhise iwe apii. Aazha niibiwa gegoon gii-ani-aanjise bimaadiziwin. Gaa-bimibizowaad ogidaagonag gii-ayaawag. Gaawiin noongom animoo' o-gii-aabaji'asiwaawaa' ininiwag gii-gii'osewaad gaye gii-bagdawaawaad. Gaawiin noongom o-gii-gichi-inenimaasiwaawaa' animoo'. Gii-babaamiba'idiwag animoshag miziwe biniskwe. Gaawiin noongom awiyag gii-bimosesiiwag. Gii-izhaawaad adaawewigamigong gii-bimibizowag odaabaanensing. Gaa-mazinaateseg gaye o-gii-ayaanaawaa. Gii-adaawaadegin adaawewigamigong gakina awiya zhemaak gii-adaawe. CBC eta gii-mazinaatese iwe apii, ango-diba'igan endaso-giizhig. Amii ko iwe apii gakina awiya gaa-gibitinang wegonen ezhichigewaad e-ando-ganawaabandamowaad gaa-mazinaatesenig.

Bezhig wiisaakodewikwe ngojigo naanimidana daso-biboone Rose o-gii-wiidanokiimaan adaawewigamigong. Apane ko wii-minikwe nibi. Wewiib ako ozhagashkinaanan mazina'iiginoonsan makakong wedi dash gaa-izhi-ayaag gaa-mookojiwang nibi izhaa eminikwed ango-minikwaagan nibi. Biizhaa ajina e-anokiid. Aazha miinawaa wii-minikwe nibi. Amii sa gabe-giizhig iwe ezhichiged e-minikwed nibi gaawiin dash debijii'aabowesii. Gegapii o-ganoonigoon bezhig owiidanokiimaaganan. Aaniish owaabamigoon bizhishig e-minikwenid nibi gaye gaawiin aapiji waabisiiwan. Odinaan

Hunters and fishermen used snowmobiles for their work and no longer ran alongside dog-pulled sleds. Many of the dogs were neither respected nor looked after. Locals didn't walk to the grocery store anymore; they drove for even the smallest errand and trucks and cars crowded the narrow streets. For the first time, the store began to stock televisions. People bought them up so quickly the store couldn't keep them stocked. CBC was the only channel in those days, and it was on for just an hour a day – but when that hour came, people all around town stopped whatever they were doing to go to their living room or the living room of someone who had a TV. And they sat immobile for an entire hour looking at the screen and watching the news.

A Métis lady, about 50 years old, worked with Rose at the store in those days, and she was thirsty. She stuck some price tickets on a stack of boxes, then hustled over to the water fountain, gulped a whole cup of water, and came back to work. One minute later, she needed to drink again. She drank and drank, all day long, but couldn't quench her thirst. Rose could see the desperation on her face, as if she would die of thirst even after having so much water, and it was something terrible. Another lady working there saw all this, and noticed too that the thirsty lady's vision had gotten much worse in ji-ando-waabamaad mashkikiiwininiwan. Onoondaan e-ayaamagak inaapinewin. Debwe gii-bigiiwe awe ikwe. Odayaan gegoon ge-aabajitood ji-jiita'odizod. Amii dash gaa-izhichiged endaso-giizhig ejiita'odizod. Amii owe ge-izhichigeyaan wii-bimaadiziyaan odigowaan. Ngoding ako gaawiin deminik iweni gii-jiita'odizod. Apatoo ko imaa gaa-izhi-ozhichigaadeg gaa-makadewaagamig, e-miijid ziizibaakwad. Amii ini miinawaa bezhig gaa-gikenimaad Rose iwe e-inaapinenid.

Amii noongom iwe inaapinewin e-maajii-dazhinjigaadeg. Niibiwa awiyag iwe inaapinewag. Rose owiijiiwaagana' gaye awiyag gaa-daawaad besho, gaye gichi-ay'aag, gaye odinawemaagana'. Bepezhig Rose oshiimeya' gaye omiseya' iwe inaapinewa'. Bezhig gii-ozhigwaapine. 1991 gii-izhisenig Rose gii-maadanokii CHR e-inanokiid. Niishtana daso-biboon apane ishkwaawaach gaa-gii-waabamaapan ini ikwezensan ejiita'odizonid. Noongom dash endaso-giizhig owaabamaa' awiya' eziizibaakwadwaapinenid. Endaso-giizis aazha miinawaa awiya wiindamawaa iwe e-inaapined, egoshkwendang dash.

a few weeks. She gently told the thirsty lady to go to the doctor – she had heard about an illness that made people thirsty and affected their eyesight. Maybe there was some medicine. A few days later, the thirsty lady was back at work with an enormous glass-and-metal syringe. She stabbed the needle into a bottle of insulin, pulled back to fill the syringe, and injected it into her flesh every single day. She would have to do this, she said, for the rest of her life. Sometimes the insulin wouldn't be enough; she would feel shaky and would run to the coffee tray and pop a sugar cube into her mouth. She was the second person with diabetes that Rose ever met.

Then, suddenly, talk of diabetes was everywhere in the community. Rose's friends and neighbours, several elders, even her family had diabetes. One by one, Rose's seven sisters were diagnosed, and one of them even had two miscarriages as a result of the disease. In 1991, Rose began working as a Community Health Representative (CHR) for the Cree Board of Health and Social Services of James Bay. Twenty years had passed since she had met the thirsty lady and thirty years since she had seen the girl with the needle in high school, and now Rose worked every day with people with diabetes. More people were being newly diagnosed every month – and almost every one of them was surprised.

"Gaawiin editawe!" ako ikidowag. "Gaawiin wiikaa nimiijisiin gaa-zhiiwang. Gaawiin iwe nindinaapinesiidog."

Owiindamawaa' idash ako, e-omashkiigomod, bakwezhigan bezhig gegoon gaa-maanishkaagemagak. Daabishkoo ziizibaakwad inendaagwan bakwezhigan.

"Nin-gichi-ayaamag o-gii-amwaawaan bakwezhiganan gaawiin dash wiikaa gii-ziizibaakwadwaapinesiiwag," ikidowag miinawaa.

"Eya," odinaa'. "O-gii-amwaawaan bakwezhiganan. Wiinge dash gaye gii-gichi-anokiiwag endaso-giizhig. Gaawiin giinawind iwe gidizhi-bimaadizisiimin noongom."

O-gii-maajii-dazhindaan ziizibaakwadwaapinewin bizinjiganing, ewiindamaaged gaawiin awiya odaa-amwaasiin waabimanoominan gaye opiniin gii-wiisinid. Ziizibaakwad inendaagwanoon ini miijiman. Giishpin ginwesh bimoseyin, gidaa-niisinaan ziizibaakwad gi-miskwiiming niizhogon. Giishpin minikweyin ishkodewaabo zhingobiiwaabo zhoominaabo wegonen igo iwe dinookaan, gaawiin onizhishinzinoon ozaam daabishkoo ziizibaakwad inendaagwan. Aapiji niibiwa noongom iwe gii-inaapinewa' gaawiin

"That can't be right," they would say to her. "I never eat sweets. It can't be diabetes."

Rose would explain to each person, in the Cree language that the doctors and nurses couldn't speak, that the flour in dumplings and bannock might not taste sweet, but it was a kind of sugar nevertheless.

"But," they would say, "our grandparents ate bannock and dumplings and they didn't have diabetes."

"Yes," Rose would answer, "they ate bannock and dumplings. But think of all the exercise they did that we don't do. Think of all the ways our lives are different from theirs."

She began talking about diabetes on the radio and in schools, teaching people not to have both rice and potatoes in the same meal because both are a kind of sugar, teaching that a long walk would lower blood sugar for up to two days, teaching that alcohol could be dense with sugar even if it didn't taste sweet, teaching that stress aggravated the disease. And still, there were so many new diagnoses of diabetes and other chronic illnesses that Rose couldn't do all the work herself and the Cree Board of Health

gii-de-izhisesii ji-wiiji'aad gakina.
Ndawaach bezhig miinawaa gii-anokii'aa.

Miinawaa dash bezhig.

Miinawaa bezhig.

Aayaakaw ako Rose gewiin gii-nanaando-gikenindizo ji-ziizibaakwadwaapinegwen. Gaawiin gii-inamanji'osii daabishkoo gaa-inamanji'owaad iwe gaa-inaapinewaad. Niibiwa dash odinawemaagana' o-gii-ayaanaawaa iwe aazha. Gii-ojaanimendam gaye nasine iwe apii giiyaabi gii-nitaa-giiwashkwebiinid onaabeman, ji-boonitoonid. Niibiwa awiyag gii-aakoziwag odazhiikewining. Ginwesh gii-mino-ayaa Rose. Obiidoonan ako iniwe gaa-aabajichigaadegin ji-gikenjigaadeg. Onanaando-gikenimaan ako onaabeman gaye oniijaanisa'. Amii noongom gaa-inanjige'aad oniijaanisa' iwe broccoli.

Aabiding dash 1997 gii-izhisenig gii-nanaando-gikenindizod, gii-ishpaakoshkaani iweni. Amii gewiin iwe ji-inaapined inendam. O-gii-maajii-odaapinaan mashkiki.Nawach gaye gii-maajii-babaamose gaye gwayak e-gagwe-inanjiged. Aabiding dash e-gizhaatenig gii-ziigwang 2002 gii-izhisenig, gii-zaaga'am imaa gaa-dananokiid. Aazha tagiin midaaso-diba'iganens gii-zaaga'amooban aazha dash miinawaa e-inamanji'od. Nanaando-gikenindizo. Wiinge ishpaakoshkaani

had to hire another CHR for Chisasibi just to meet the demand.

And then another.

And then another.

From time to time, Rose used the glucose-testing kits to screen herself. She didn't have diabetes symptoms, but it ran in her family and there was quite a bit of stress in her home in those days, before her husband stopped drinking. So many people in the community were getting sick. For years her test results were fine but Rose continued self-screening. For years, she brought test kits home from work and tested her husband and all her kids. She even did what she had vowed never to do: she made her children eat broccoli – but without even once using the extreme residential school methods.

One day, in '97, her self-screening showed a new result: pre-diabetes, a warning sign that diabetes was not far away. Rose began to take medication and became still more diligent about exercise and careful eating. Then, on a sunny day in spring 2002, she went to the bathroom at work and remembered, as she zipped up her pants, that she had been to the bathroom just ten minutes earlier – and ten minutes before that. She could already feel she would need the toilet in a few minutes again. She crossed the office to the

9

iweni. Amii sa gewiin Rose Swallow eziizibaakwadwaapined.

Wiinge gichi-ikwanaamo. Bagidanaamo. Apane miinawaa izhaa imaa zaaga'amoowigamigong.

Giiyaabi iwe inanokii Rose imaa Jizaasibiing. Aazha naananiwag iwe gaa-inanokiiwaad. Wiin odazhiikaan e-gikino'amaaged aaniin ge-izhichigeng giishpin ziizibaakwadwaapineyin. Gakina gaa-ayaawaad imaa Jizaasibiing odookishkaagonaawaa iwe inaapinewin. Aazha gaye nawach ani-oshkaadiziwag iwe gaa-inaapinewaad. Amii dash ezhichiged Rose e-wiiji'aad awiya' ji-gojitoowaad ini gitigaanan wiikaa gaa-gii-miijisigwaa gaa-onizhishingin ji-miijinaaniwangin. Izhichige ji-gojipidamowaad jibwaa-adaawewaad adaawewigamigong. Amii gaye ezhichiged e-wiindamawaad awiya' ji-mitosenid, gaawiin ji-bimibizosigwaa miziwe. Odinaa' gaye ji-gagwejiinid. Amii dash enaagwak noongom imaa Jizaasibiing, e-gagwejiiwaad awiyag gagwejiiwigamigong gaye ebimosewaad miikanaang gemaa jiigew ziibiing gii-niibininig, gaye ebabaamaagimosewaad gii-biibooninig. Gaamashi awiyan

cupboard with the test kits. She pricked her finger with the lancet, wiped the blood on the strip, and inserted it into the reader. The number in the glucose reader was too high. Rose Swallow, like the needle girl in high school and the thirsty lady from the Hudson's Bay Store, like every one of her sisters, had diabetes.

She sucked in a deep breath and let it out. And then she ran back to the bathroom.

Rose is still a CHR in Chisasibi, along with four other CHRs. She's in charge of the diabetes portfolio and spends most of her work time teaching people, in their own language, how to manage the disease. By now, every Chisasibi family is directly affected by diabetes and the newly diagnosed are getting younger and younger. Rose organizes healthy-food tastings. Vegetables and fruits are so expensive in the North that people don't want to spend money on new ones they might not like, so Rose finds ways to let them taste new foods without having to pay all that money. She also organizes Leave-Your-Vehicle-At-Home days for people to try exercising as a way of getting to work, as their grandparents once did. And she encourages people to try the fitness centre, even if it is a little intimidating at first. Chisasibi is seeing big changes again: people are exercising more, walking outside along the highway owaabamaasiin ji-bimibatoonid animoo' gii-odaaba'iwenid daabishkoo gaa-gii-nitaa-izhichigenid omishoomisan.

Daabishkoo gakina ini gaa-gikino'amawaad Rose, amii gewiin ezhichiged e-odaapinaad omashkikiima' endaso-giizhig, gaye e-nanaando-gikendang omiskwiim. Omiijinan gitigaanensan gaye ozaawi-manoominan ogiizizwaan. Gaawiin gaye gagwe-ojaanimendanzii. Giishpin ojaanimendang aapiji wiiba ishpaagoshkaani gaa-aabajitood ji-gikendang ezhisenig omiskwiim. Amii ko ezhi-gichi-babaapagidanaamod nishikaach. Gemaa odagindaan mazina'igan gaa-zaagitood. Noongom gaye gaawiin minikwesiiwan onaabeman. Noongom oniijaanisa' gaye oozhisa' gaa-ojaanimendami'igod. Ngoding oganawenimaa' oozhisa' giishpin naganaaganiwinid. Aapiji ko ojaanimendam iwe gii-izhisenig.

Amii ko egod onaabeman, "Haaw sa, Rose, aazha gidoojaanimendam gidizhinaagoz. Ando-babaamosedaa."

Wawepizowag dash gaye owawepinaawaa' oozhisiwaa' ozaam egisinaanig agwajiing, apane dash e-ando-babaamosewaad miikwanaang, ewaasaagonagaag gaa-izhi-ishpadaasing, e-babaamaagonagiinid oozhisiwaa'.

or the river in the long summer evenings, or snowshoeing across the open spaces in winter. So far, though, Rose hasn't seen anyone running alongside a dog team.

Like all the people she teaches, Rose has to work at her own diabetes every day. She takes her pills and tests her blood sugar. She experiments with vegetables and cooks with whole grains and high fibre. She has to be especially careful about stress – it's the one thing drives up her blood sugar levels very quickly. Sometimes calming down is as easy as taking a few deep breaths or reading a good book. Years ago, her husband's drinking was what drove up her anxiety, but he hasn't had a drink in years. These days, Rose worries for her kids and grandkids and also looks after some of her grandkids on the days they're neglected. It gets to be a lot of work and anxiety for someone no longer young enough to sit on her grandfather's dogsled.

Then her husband says, "Oh Rosie. I can see on your face – it's time to go for a walk."

And they tie on their boots and swaddle the grandkids against the cold and head out for a long walk by the highway where the sun glints off the snowdrifts and the grandkids kick up snow around them.